Confronting and Overcoming Arthritis

Confronting and Overcoming Arthritis

✦

A guide to the emotional challenges of illness

Rev. Warren H. Seyfert

Illustrations by Ralph Seyfert

iUniverse, Inc.
New York Lincoln Shanghai

Confronting and Overcoming Arthritis
A guide to the emotional challenges of illness

iUniverse books may be ordered through booksellers or by contacting:

iUniverse
2021 Pine Lake Road, Suite 100
Lincoln, NE 68512
www.iuniverse.com
1-800-Authors (1-800-288-4677)

Because of the dynamic nature of the Internet, any Web addresses or links contained in this book may have changed since publication and may no longer be valid.

This book is not intended to be a substitute for medical care of people with arthritis, and treatment should not be based solely on its contents. Instead, treatment must be developed in a dialogue between the individual and the treating physician. This book has been written to help with that dialogue.

ISBN: 978-0-595-47850-7 (pbk)
ISBN: 978-0-595-60103-5 (ebk)

Printed in the United States of America

DEDICATED

TO MY WIFE

RUTH

AND OUR CHILDREN

DAVID
PETER
NANCY
CAROL

Contents

FOREWORD

Confronting and Overcoming Arthritis is a treatise on learning to live with disabling physical problems. Warren Seyfert, a minister of Christian faith, confronted rheumatoid arthritis. He planned to function, survive, and live with progressive disability.

In this book he has presented ways to succeed in living with disabilities. Warren Seyfert has outlined the feelings one must confront, identifying the psychological concepts necessary to experience life rather than to just exist in life. Life with physical disabilities must be planned while cultivating humor, enduring frustration, combating depression, and accepting reality. Determining priorities and developing an outlook that allows ultimate function is a large part of the plan.

All who read this message of hope from Reverend Seyfert must inspect themselves, inspect their struggle to survive emotionally and physically, and benefit from the real confrontation with their feelings. That will insure that they indeed will live.

Dean A. Hauter, M.D.
Abraham Lincoln Medical Group
Lincoln, Illinois

PREFACE

A person's adjustment to having a chronic disease is always difficult. Control of these diseases usually requires a discipline of medications and dietary or physical limitations. People with arthritic diseases have an additional burden. Arthritis limits physical activity—often even ordinary ambulation or personal functions. Perhaps even more important—arthritis (especially rheumatoid arthritis) attacks a person's body image. For all these reasons, denial, anger, frustration, and depression are common among arthritis sufferers.

For the physician, comprehensive treatment of arthritis consists of as precise a diagnosis as possible, establishment of stage or degree of disease, and prescription of medications and physical and occupational therapy. In addition, physicians try to help patients understand their arthritic disease. We know the problems they face. However, enlightened patients are more effective than professionals in helping themselves and other arthritis sufferers cope with their emotional struggle.

Reverend Seyfert, who himself has severe rheumatoid arthritis, has approached the problem of coping and adjusting in this volume. He carefully enumerates the stages of human response upon acquiring arthritis—the anger, denial, frustration, and depression. Throughout the chapters, he deals with these human responses and offers some positive recommendations for other patients. Without being unrealistic, he suggests a variety of techniques to once again gain reasonable control of the direction of one's life, even with an impairing arthritic disease. He suggests expressing emotions instead of containing them; sharing problems; assuming responsibility; and relying upon humor. Physicians diagnose disease and recommend therapies, but patients must assume responsibility in the implementation of therapeutic regimens, at least in chronic diseases like arthritis. He has found these techniques useful in maintaining self-esteem and thus minimizing depression. His own reflections obviously are self-serving, but in that process perhaps equally useful to millions of others who have difficulty living with arthritis. This may be more useful to our patients than many of the kind words and life style recommendations made by us—the treating physicians.

Gerson C. Bernhard, M.D.
Medical Director
Midwest Arthritis Treatment Center

Clinical Professor of Medicine
Medical College of Wisconsin

1

CONFRONTING ARTHRITIS

"To You, O Goddess of Efficiency,
Your happy vassals bend the reverent knee,
Save when arthritis, your benighted foe,
Sulks in the bones, and sourly mumbles "No!"

—Samuel Hoffenstein

Every year, one million people will learn that they have arthritis. It was at the age of forty-two years that I was informed by my family physician that he had arrived at an early diagnosis of rheumatoid arthritis, and his opinion was later verified with further testing at the Illinois Research Hospital in Chicago.

Many men and women—from childhood to old age—are afflicted with some form or degree of arthritis. The Arthritis Foundation estimates that more than thirty-six million Americans—one in every seven—have some type of arthritis. About 250,000 children have juvenile arthritis. Women are more prone to arthritis than men, the onset usually occurring during the thirties or forties, but some forms developing during the later years, along with the aging process.

WARNING SIGNS

Arthritis is defined as inflammation of the joints. Arth = joint + itis = inflammation. Warning signs are the swelling of any joint, inability to move a joint properly, or unexplained weight loss, fever, or weakness combined with joint pain.

Arthritis is part of a larger group called rheumatic diseases. There are more than one hundred types of arthritis, the most common of which are rheumatoid arthritis, osteoarthritis, systemic lupus erythematosus, scleroderma, and gout. Other forms are juvenile arthritis, ankylosing, spondylitis, psoriatic arthritis, infectious arthritis, fibrositis, bursitis, and tendonitis.

CAUSE AND CURE UNKNOWN

Neither the cause nor the cure of arthritis is known at this time, although there are several theories, and considerable research is being done. Most forms of arthritis are chronic, alternating between flare-ups and remissions, but often lasting for a lifetime. Understandably, anyone suffering from arthritis seeks to find relief from the pain and stiffness and immobility. Consequently, arthritics are the most exploited group of people with health problems in our society. Television commercials continually barrage us with the promise of quick relief from the minor pains of arthritis. It is estimated that almost one billion dollars are spent each year on worthless drugs, diets, devices, or clinics. Many of these have harmful effects because they delay proper medical treatment.

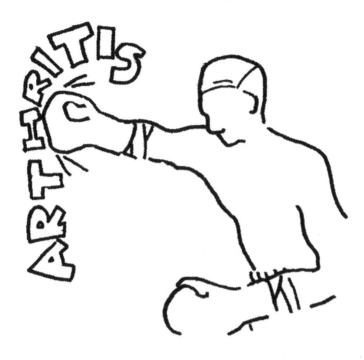

Confronting Arthritis

IMPORTANCE OF EARLY TREATMENT

Early treatment is essential, since damage done by arthritis is often irreversible. Individual programs of preventive care need to be worked out under the supervision of a rheumatologist or a physician who understands the nature of the disease. Much of the danger of over-the-counter drugs is that they delay early diagnosis and treatment until it is too late to prevent damage to the joints.

Arthritis can be very deceptive. Sometimes the use of quack cures is coincidental with a remission. Also, during remission, there is a tendency to discontinue prescribed medications. Do not be deceived. Enjoy a remission to the utmost, but don't forget, you still have arthritis.

There are excellent books available that can help you to understand your disease better. Much valuable literature is available from the Arthritis Foundation, which may have a local chapter in your area. My purpose is not to discuss the medical aspects of arthritis, but to share some of the experiences I have had in living with arthritis.

MAINTAIN A HEALTHY OUTLOOK

When my doctor first diagnosed my arthritis, he made the statement that "You can't get arthritis of the brain." Though we may suffer from a sick body, we can maintain a healthy mind. Since we are thinking beings, we can reason our way through any situation. You, too, can think of ways to adjust to living with your arthritis.

Because I have lived with arthritis for the past twenty years, I believe that my own experiences may offer some help and hope to others who may be similarly afflicted. Essentially, the message that I have to share is that the real answer to coping with the knowledge that we have an incurable disease is in learning how to live with arthritis with proper medical help, and not in seeking some miracle cure. Difficult as it is to face up to this reality, it is possible for you to overcome physical limitations through positive psychological attitudes. You must first accept the hard fact that you have arthritis before you can learn to live with its effects.

The following chapters in this book contain insights I have gained from living with arthritis. My hope in sharing these observations is that you, the reader, may find some encouragement and hope from a fellow sufferer.

WE ARE IN GOOD COMPANY

We can be assured that we are not alone. We are in good company with Alexander the Great, Julius Caesar, Henry VIII, John Milton, Martin Luther, Pierre Renoir, Queen Victoria, Christopher Columbus, Benjamin Franklin, Mark Twain, Bing Crosby, Rosalind Russell, Joe Nameth, Johnny Bench, Arnold Palmer, Henry Fonda, Elvis Presley, Eric Sevareid, Betty Ford, Barry Goldwater, Rose Kennedy, Agatha Christie, and Dr. Christian Barnard.

2

FEELING IMPRISONED

"But though my wing is closely bound,
My heart's at liberty.
My prison walls cannot control
The flight, the freedom of my soul."

—Jeanne Guyon

"The Prisoner's Dream" (Traum des Gefangenen) by the artist Moritz von Schwind is displayed in the Schack Gallery in Munich, Germany. The subject depicted by the painter is escape. The gnomes standing one above the other represent the successive positions to be assumed in climbing up to the window. The features of the gnome at the top appear to resemble those of the prisoner, who is himself filing through the prison bars.

Any arthritis sufferer shares "The Prisoner's Dream" that somehow he or she can escape the narrow limits that have been imposed. One seeks some window that admits a ray of light in the midst of a difficult situation.

EVEN THE CAGED BIRD SINGS

Anyone who suffers from arthritis can understand how the limitations of the body threaten to imprison the freedom of the spirit. There is a yearning to be liberated from the pain, discomfort, and immobility of the body. Like a bird in a cage, one feels confined, haunted by the question, "Can the caged bird sing?"

The Greek philosopher Plato described the body as the prison of the soul. He regarded the body as an impediment, which limited and imprisoned the soul. As arthritics, we, too, can appreciate the conflict between the limitations of the body and the desire of the soul, or spirit, to be set free.

Every prisoner needs to have a dream. But, alas, dreams are not reality. And though a victim of arthritis may dream of escaping from the body's imprisoning limits, during this life the spirit continues to reside in the body.

Like a prisoner serving his sentence, you may be inclined to ask such questions as these: "Do I deserve this? Have I done something wrong? Why am I being punished? Should I feel guilty?" There is a great temptation to blame ourselves for what has happened, with the result that we feel sorry for ourselves.

CHOOSING ONE'S ATTITUDE

Viktor Frankl, who was unjustly committed to a German concentration camp during World War II, expressed many of his thoughts in a remarkable book called <u>Man's Search For Meaning</u>. One of his observations was that "the last of human freedoms is the ability to choose one's attitude in a given set of circumstances."[1]

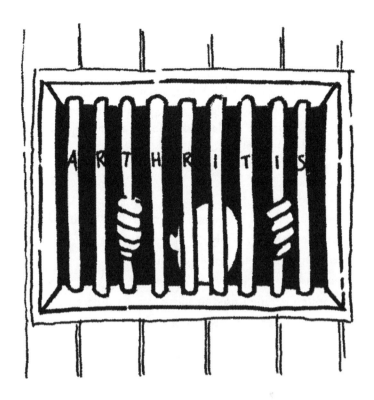

Feeling Imprisoned

We may not be able to change the situation in which we find ourselves, but we can determine our attitude toward our condition. One young woman, faced with an incurable illness, expressed her feelings in this way: "It's not what happens to you, but what you do about it, that makes the difference."

Some of the world's most profound literature was written by people in prison. John Bunyan penned his famous <u>Pilgrim's Progress</u>; Saint Paul wrote most of his letters in the New Testament while under house arrest; Dietrich Bonhoeffer's writings are collected in <u>his Letters and Papers From Prison</u>. In his poetic lines, "Who Am I?" Bonhoeffer describes his inner struggle:

> Who am I?
> They often tell me I stepped from my cell's confinement
> Calmly, cheerfully, firmly,
> Like a squire from his country-house.
> Who am I?
> They often tell me I used to speak to my warders
> As though it were mine to command.
> Who am I?
> They also tell me I bore the days of misfortune
> Equably, smilingly, proudly,
> Like one accustomed to win.
> Am I then really all that which other men tell of?
> Or am I only what I myself know of myself?
> Restless and longing and sick, like a bird in a cage,
> Struggling for breath, as though hands were compressing my throat,
> Yearning for colors, for flowers, for the voices of birds,
> Thirsting for words of kindness, for neighborliness,
> Tossing in expectation of great events,
> Powerfully trembling for friends at an infinite distance,
> Weary and empty at praying, at thinking, at making,
> Faint, and ready to say farewell to it all?
> Who am I? This or the other?
> Am I one person today and tomorrow another?
> Am I both at once? A hypocrite before others,
> And before myself a contemptible woebegone weakling?

Or is something within me still like a beaten army,

Fleeing in disorder from victory already achieved?

Who am I? They mock me, these lonely questions of mine.[2]

FREEDOM TO CHOOSE

There are a number of ways in which we can react to the situations in which we find ourselves:

We can deny that a bad situation exists. Our first response is likely to be: "This isn't really happening."

We can pretend that the situation isn't there—a kind of hide and seek game. We can run away and hide from life's problems and difficulties, hoping they won't catch up with us.

We can rebel, get angry with everyone for conspiring against us.

We can resign ourselves to the situation and not do anything about it, giving up and yielding to our condition.

Or, we can determine that we will find ways to overcome our situation and become victors instead of victims. Like the prisoner who wrote on the wall of his cell the words: "It is not adversity that kills, but the manner in which we bear adversity."

Although it is possible to confine the body, nothing can imprison the human spirit. Although we often cannot change our situation, we can change the way we feel about it. The limitations of the body cannot restrict the freedom of the spirit. You, too, have the capacity to choose what your attitude will be toward your arthritis.

"Two men looked out through prison bars.

One saw mud; the other saw stars."

3

ACCEPTING LIMITATIONS

"God grant me the serenity to accept
The things I cannot change,
Courage to change the things I can,
And wisdom to know the difference."

—Reinhold Niebuhr

Most people take for granted their ability to walk, to run, to dance. People find pleasure in hiking, biking, jogging, bowling, golfing, and skiing. It is a severe shock to find that because of arthritis—or other disabilities—serious limitations are imposed upon one's ability to function. A homemaker discovers that using the vacuum, making beds, or working in the garden are increasingly difficult. A workman finds that he can no longer carry out his duties as a mechanic, construction worker, or machine operator.

WHAT'S HAPPENING TO ME?

Deformed feet make it difficult to keep one's balance; misshapen ankles make walking painful; arthritic knees make climbing stairs a problem; stiff hips cause embarrassment when trying to get up from a chair; aching elbows eliminate bowling from among one's recreational activities; and weak wrists make simple tasks difficult. Gradually, one by one, the things we enjoyed doing, or had learned to do for a living, are no longer possible.

We experience feelings of anger and envy toward those who can still do things and take them so much for granted. There is a sense of self-pity: "Why did this happen to me? How can I possibly accept these limitations?"

Without realizing it, we are going through a grief experience—with its stages of denial, anger, resentment, guilt, and eventually, acceptance. But it is a long, agonizing process. While we are going through it, there seems to be no end, and no way of knowing where we will come out. Often there appears to be no light at the end of the tunnel. When others try to counsel us, we become hostile. "How can they possibly know how we feel? How can they understand what it means to accept limitations?"

GAINING A NEW PERSPECTIVE

No one else can really tell us how to accept our situation. Acceptance comes, not from outside ourselves, but from within. It is not others, but we ourselves, who must grapple with our limitations and determine what our attitude is to be toward them.

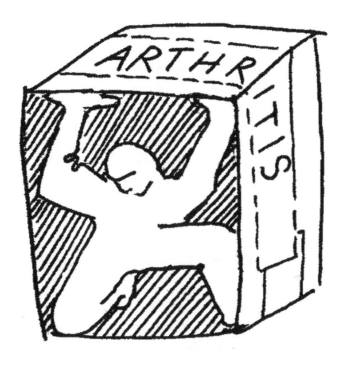

Accepting Limitations

Our natural tendency is to focus on the things we can no longer do. What we have lost seems to outweigh any possible gains. But the secret of living with our limitations is to evaluate the things we can still do. Instead of seeing our glass of water as half-empty, we need to come to the awareness that it is still half-full. It is a matter of gaining a new perspective on our lives, learning to maximize the abilities we do have, rather than lamenting what we do not have. Disabled persons develop the ability to make the best possible use of their remaining abilities and skills.

People seem to grow stronger through adversity than they do amid prosperity. Easy times tend to soften us up; hard times can make us tougher. This is not necessarily so, but the possibility is there. Nor is this to say that suffering is a good thing. It is not that suffering causes us to develop endurance. But it can, and often does, produce a determination to be victors, rather than victims. Bad weather does not cause good weather; but good weather often follows bad weather.

NO SITUATION IS EVER HOPELESS

Accepting limitations does not come easily. For some of us, it may not come at all. It all depends upon whether we can bring forth the inner strength to make the most of a bad situation. Life confronts us with two choices—despair or hope. Despair is the easy way out. Hope is difficult to come by, but it is the only positive solution. There is no hopeless situation—it is only our reaction that makes our situation appear hopeless. In your life, and in mine, hope can win out over despair.

My own experience is that acceptance is never a once-and-for-all decision. One can find his or her situation acceptable today, and not far down the road confront the same struggle again. Perhaps, like any other bad news, we cannot fully comprehend its impact at a given moment. It can only be assimilated by degrees, a little at a time. But each fragment that we grasp makes us better able to lay hold of the next. Dealing with the future is built upon the struggles and victories of the past. Because we faced up to yesterday, the possibility and probability is great that we can also face up to today, and, when the time comes, tomorrow.

4

HANDLING FRUSTRATION

"Difficulties are meant to rouse, not discourage.
The human spirit is to grow strong by conflict."

—William Ellery Channing

Life is a mysterious mixture of success and failure, joy and sorrow, accomplishment and disappointment. We welcome the good things that happen to us, but resent the misfortunes. We feel good when things are going well for us, but we become easily discouraged by obstacles to our happiness.

Sometimes it is not so much the big things that trouble us as it is the petty, minor irritations. We may have the courage and motivation to face crises, but become frustrated over our inability to accomplish small tasks. Opening a milk carton, pulling a zipper, or getting a button through a buttonhole can infuriate and frustrate one, as countless efforts continue to be unsuccessful. The final, angry reaction is "The hell with it!"

SOME FALSE ASSUMPTIONS

Any arthritic immediately understands this sense of deep frustration. The harder one tries, the worse it gets. Why must such simple, trivial tasks be so difficult, when others do them without thinking? Why must everything be such a tremendous effort?

In her carefully researched book, Physical Disability: A Psychosocial Approach, Beatrice Wright, of the University of Kansas, examines some of the studies that have been done regarding frustration. There are two common assumptions that are challenged by evidence to the contrary. One assumption is that persons with disabilities are more frequently frustrated than the non-disabled. The other assumption is that persons with a disability react more immaturely to frustrating situations confronting them, that they are more irritable and easily frustrated. Studies show both of these assumptions to be false. Furthermore, contrary to expectations, studies conducted among children showed few differences between those handicapped and those non-handicapped children to frustrating situations.

Author Beatrice Wright examines what she refers to as "myths" about the relationship between physical disabilities and frustration.

1) The outsider views the situation of another in the way he imagines he would feel in a like situation.

2) The outsider tends to be unfamiliar with the ways of circumventing difficulties.

3) The outsider perceives disability as a negative state and perceives frustration connected with the disability as especially frustrating.

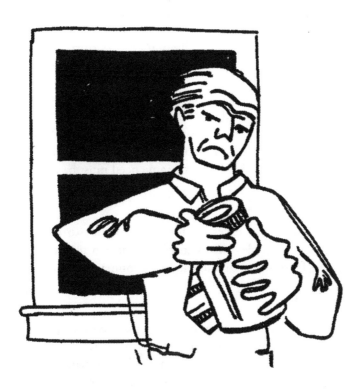

Handling Frustrations

4)   The outsider perceives disability as so central a cause that it is held account-
       able for unrelated events in the life of the disabled person.

5)   The outsider's expectation that disability causes frustration serves his biases
       and assumptions, causing him to see what he wants to see.[3]

What is overlooked in all these "myths" is the truth that frustration can, and
often does, lead to learning and growth. The negative effects of frustration tend
to be emphasized, and the positive by-products are often overlooked. The significant factor, when our activities are blocked, is to use our energies constructively.
New goals and alternatives that meet the same need must be discovered, and thus
our ingenuity is challenged.

Beatrice Wright concludes that:

> The value of reducing excessive frustration is not to eliminate frustration
> from the lives of people, but to enable the person to deal with and learn to
> tolerate new frustrations that inevitably accompany new challenges.[4]

HANG IN THERE

It seems that arthritics are generally stubborn, persistent people, who do not give
up easily. It is not entirely clear whether we are basically that way by temper-
ament, or whether we become that way from dealing with our arthritis. But in
either case, that obstinacy is at the same time the source of both our endurance
and our frustration. We are determined to "hang in there" and "fight one more
round."

Family members and friends, sensing our irritation, seek to be of help. Perhaps
the greatest mistake made by loved ones is not that they do too little, but that
they do too much. Faced with frustration, it is too easy for us to accept a helping
hand, to become overly dependent upon those who are all too willing to assist us
in our efforts. The invalid who dominates the household like a tyrant may well
have become that way because caring people were too willing to help.

SELF-HELP IS BEST

Faced with offers of help, my own response has always been: "Let me try it
myself, and if I need help, I'll ask for it." There are times when assistance must be
graciously accepted and welcomed, but only after our own efforts have failed.
There is nothing wrong with failure; our only error is in not having tried. It is
through trial and error that we develop alternatives. By using our ingenuity, we
learn how to outsmart frustrating situations.

In addition to using our own resourcefulness, considerable aid can be found in the <u>Self-Help Manual for Arthritis Patients</u>, available from the Arthritis Foundation. Many helpful devices are described which simplify daily tasks for arthritis sufferers.

TAKE TIME TO UNWIND

For persons afflicted with arthritis, frustration must be converted from a negative to a positive experience. How we handle frustration has much to do with overcoming arthritis.

One of the insights that I have gained is that it is helpful to take a break after several attempts have failed. Instead of experiencing growing frustration, the secret is in taking time to unwind. Then, strangely enough, when you return to the task it usually goes quite easily. It is not the jobs to be done, but the frustration in trying to do them, that overwhelms us.

I seriously doubt that anyone with arthritis, or anyone else, for that matter, ever completely conquers feelings of discouragement and frustration. But we can learn how to work around such feelings and get things done, no matter how difficult they may be. And, if all else fails, we can be thankful if we are fortunate enough to have caring family members and friends to do the things for us that we cannot do for ourselves.

5

MASTERING DEPRESSION

"We must never despair; our situation has been compromising before, and it has changed for the better; so I trust it will again. If new difficulties arise, we must put forth new exertion and proportion our efforts to the exigencies of the times."

—George Washington

Life is made up of mountains, valleys, and plateaus. At times we climb the heights, or sink to the depths, or walk on level places. One cannot always remain on the high places of joy or success, but neither should we continue too long in the low places of sorrow or despair. Even though we walk through valleys, we are not meant to stay there permanently. Much of our life is lived on the plateaus of routine, ordinary activity.

Someone observed wisely that life is like an elevator, with its ups and downs. Hopefully, each person finds that there are more ups than downs. My own experience has been that, when we add up life's pluses and minuses, there are more pluses than minuses.

TURNING ANGER INSIDE OUT

Everyone gets depressed at times. No person is able to be in good spirits continually. So long as our mood swings are not too extreme, or do not persist for prolonged periods, we are not unusual.

Unfortunately, for those of us who suffer from arthritis, one of the side-effects is depression. We are inclined to compare what we are no longer able to do with what we formerly did. The passing of years reduces for everyone the physical abilities, but for arthritics such limitations are especially conducive to moods of depression and hopelessness.

It has been suggested that depression is our reaction when we are unable to express anger. There is little doubt that being afflicted with arthritis makes us angry. It is difficult to know where to direct our anger, but when it is unexpressed, it turns inward upon ourselves. One of the unresolved questions is how to express anger constructively. All around us we see too many examples of anger expressed destructively through violence and anti-social behavior. It is a continuing challenge to discover acceptable channels for displaying anger.

While we are feeling depressed, the important thing is to refrain from taking any kind of desperate action. Decisions need to be delayed until we are in a more customary frame of mind. Depressed people often take drastic steps that they would never consider taking in ordinary circumstances. So, if you find yourself depressed, delay making decisions. Wait until you come back up out of the valley.

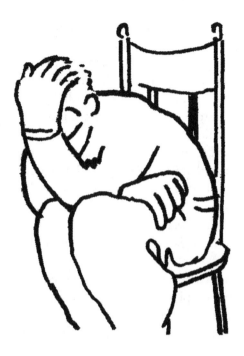

Mastering Depression

ANTI-DEPRESSANTS—GOOD OR BAD?

As the years went by, and I experienced times of depression, my doctor prescribed anti-depressants (energizers), assuring me that using them was not a sign of weakness or inability to cope, but rather represented a chemical imbalance in my body. Subsequently, I found that a carefully monitored prescription of anti-depressants helped me to maintain a healthy psychological attitude toward my arthritis. This need proved to be 'temporary, and it is no longer necessary for me to make use of this medication.

Most depression related to arthritis is reactive, that is, the illness is the reason for the unhappiness. Since there is presently no known cure for most forms of arthritis, it is understandable that people diagnosed with the disease may, at least initially, experience feelings of futility and hopelessness. But there is much that can be done to help arthritics lead a relatively normal life. The reality is not as bad as our fears of it. Arthritis is something that we can learn to live with. You can, too.

Activity is better than idleness when we are depressed. Idleness is conducive to self-pity, whereas activity occupies our minds and often helps to lift us up out of our depression. It is important to remember, however, that if depression continues for too long and becomes intensified, it may be necessary to seek professional help.

6

TOLERATING PAIN

"Pain provides an opportunity for heroism;
The opportunity is seized with surprising frequency."

—R. Harvard, M. D.

It is night. As these words are being written, I am feeling a great deal of pain. It is another one of those sleepless nights, when there seems to be no way to relieve the sharp, nagging pain. There is a loneliness about pain. Others may try to help, to understand, and to sympathize, but pain is only real to the person who is experiencing it.

After all the pain relievers and medications have been taken, after all efforts to get on top of the situation have failed, after all the tears have been shed, after all the prayers have been said, the sufferer is left alone in his misery.

PAIN TAKES PRIORITY

One cries out "Why?" but no answer comes. One asks "Is it I?" feeling that a stronger person might be better able to tolerate the pain. Others may even imply that the pain is psychological, that somehow one does not have the right attitude. But, when all is said and done, pain is very real to the sufferer.

It is difficult, although not impossible, to function while experiencing pain. Perhaps you are a person who must go to work day after day in spite of pain. Somehow, having responsibilities to carry out enables us to forget our discomfort, and, in a sense, to rise above it. Pain takes priority, unless some other activity takes on a higher priority. Work, however difficult to do, may actually free us from becoming prisoners of pain. These words, while they were being written, represent an effort to displace pain, and, for the moment at least, were successful in doing so. This book is not intended to offer easy answers. Those who suffer pain know that there are no easy answers—only hard questions. If there is a word of advice to be offered, it is that, under the stress of pain, we do nothing drastic or desperate. One needs to struggle to keep a perspective on life. The dark nights of anguish must not be allowed to blind our eyes to the bright skies of joy and hope. Tomorrow may or may not be better, but each new day provides us with the opportunity to draw strength for the road ahead. Each experience of suffering carries with it the possibility of making us stronger, better able to bear the next burden when it comes.

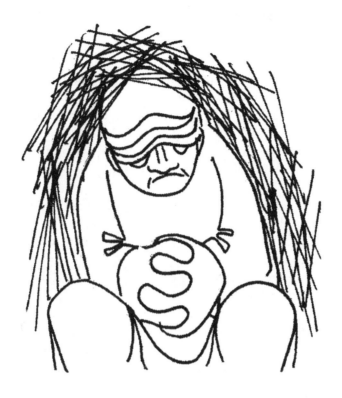

Tolerating Pain

WINNERS OR LOSERS?

You have, no doubt, cried out, as I have "How much pain can I tolerate?" Certainly we feel, at times, pushed to the edge of our limits. And yet, human beings, people like you and me, have a remarkable capacity to endure seemingly impossible situations. It is a dramatic testimony to the human spirit that women and men, and, yes, children, have been able to tolerate, even triumph over, insuperable obstacles. There is, in fact, a challenge in suffering. One hopes to be a winner, rather than a loser. One strives to be heroic, rather than cowardly. And it is this determination that "We shall overcome" that sustains us during the long nights of pain.

It is much easier to theorize about pain when one is not feeling it. We simply cannot be objective about pain while we are experiencing it. The French surgeon, Rene Leriche, once observed that "There is only one pain that is easy to bear, and that is the pain of others."

There is nothing new about pain. Primitive people asked the same questions that are in our minds today. In ancient times, people attributed pain to evil spirits which entered their bodies to torment them. Through rituals and sacrifices, efforts were made to humor or placate these unwelcome spirits.

This view eventually gave way to the idea that, whatever happened to people, they must deserve. Suffering was seen as man's destiny in life. Although these attempted explanations did not remove the pain, they served to provide the endurance and fortitude to go on living.

ALL IS NOT WELL IN THE BODY

The history of people's efforts to understand pain serves to make us aware that we are not the only ones, or the first ones, to suffer. Much as pain tends to isolate us from those who appear to be free from pain, at the same time it can also unite us with others who are experiencing pain. There is a kind of fellowship of suffering, a mutual sharing of one another's pains, which enables us to offer encouragement and hope to one another. Every one of us has been inspired and strengthened by the example of another sufferer whose endurance renewed our courage.

Although pain is physical at the outset, our emotions become quickly involved. Pain is an important defense mechanism of the body, a warning signal, indicating that something is wrong.

> We feel pain only after the pain message has traveled from the point of irritation to the brain. The pain message travels along a network of nerves to the

spinal chord and finally up to the brain. Then, when the pain message is interpreted by the brain, pain is actually felt as a body sensation.[5]

What makes pain so difficult to understand is the fact that each person has a different "pain threshold," that is, the point at which pain is perceived. Some people, for whatever reason, seem to be able to tolerate more intense pain than others.

RELIEVING SYMPTOMS OR REMOVING CAUSE?

As a nation, we Americans seem to fear pain more than anything else. To a large extent, the medical profession has become a pain-relieving industry. Pharmaceutical companies thrive on providing pain relievers. Victims of pain are exploited by all kinds of opportunists promising relief.

The problem with pain relievers is that they treat a symptom—pain—rather than the cause of the pain. It can actually be dangerous to remove pain without seeking the problem that triggers the pain.

Not enough has been done to research the problem of pain. Partly this is due to the difficulty of measuring scientifically and objectively data that is subjective in nature. However, more attention is now being given to the management of pain. Hopefully, new light can be shed upon what has troubled humans since the beginning of time.

7

CULTIVATING PATIENCE

"Patience is the best remedy for any trouble."

—Plautus (200 B.C.)

A cartoon pictured a child kneeling beside his bed in prayer, saying: "Last night I prayed for patience. What's taking so long?" Patience is a quality in short supply for most of us. We want what we want, when we want it, and we do not like to wait very long. Much of our anxiety today is geared to the instant, immediate gratification of our wishes. Impatience may be more characteristic of the young, but even as we grow older, our capacity for endurance is very limited.

The Frenchman, de Tocqueville, observed a century ago that Americans are so restless and impatient that they have invented a chair, the rocker, which enables them to be moving even when they are sitting down. Someone judged that more lives are destroyed by impatience than by any other weakness.

A SIGN OF MATURITY

It is significant that, when we are hospitalized, we are referred to as "patients." We are then in the position of waiting until nurses have time to respond to our needs. Even with the best of nursing care, it is difficult to be patient while waiting for someone to do the things we would normally do for ourselves.

It is usually others, not in our situation, who advise us to have patience. Although we have probably given that bit of wisdom to others, we find it hard to apply to ourselves.

Patience is a quality that we strive for, but never fully achieve. We only succeed, at best, in becoming less impatient. The capacity to tolerate delays and disappointments is a sign of maturity in our relationships with others, with ourselves, and with life's twists and turns. Patience involves being less critical in our judgments of others, in our evaluation of ourselves, and in our acceptance of what life measures out to us.

It is becoming increasingly evident that many health problems are related to stress, tension, and the pressures of modern society. It is difficult to avoid being caught up in this accelerated way of life. None of us seems to have the ability to slow down our pace until we are forced to do so. Few things bring us to an abrupt halt as arthritis or other physical limitations can do.

WE ALL NEED TO SLOW DOWN

I have conducted a simple survey of people's reactions to my entering an elevator while using either a cane or a wheelchair. When I apologize for being slow, the usual response is: "That's OK, we all need to slow down anyway."

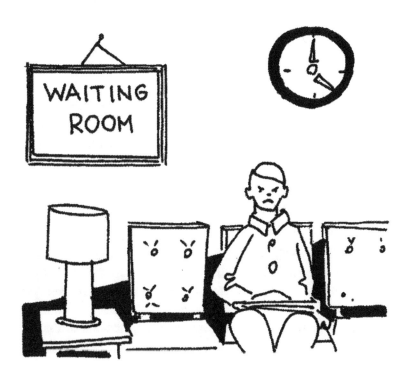

Cultivating Patience

Patience is often viewed as just stoically putting up with unwelcome situations. It might be expressed in terms of "What else can I do?" However, there is more to real patience than just putting up with one's lot in life. Patience is a quiet waiting for something to happen, a sense of expectation, not unrelated to faith and hope.

Patience exerts a quieting influence upon troubled waters. Somehow quietness and endurance sustain us in times of misfortune, whereas, in contrast, impatience and irritation can be our undoing. Patience, then, takes on a positive and constructive quality that may not change our situation but enables us to change our attitude toward our circumstances. By effecting inner transformation, somehow our outward surroundings can be viewed in a new, more promising perspective.

WHY DO PEOPLE SUFFER?

We often hear of the patience of Job, that Bible personality who suffered such great adversities. When reading the book of Job, one is more impressed by his impatience and frustration in asking the questions "Why?" and "Why me?" In seeking an answer to the question of why people suffer, the writer concludes that, although there have been various theories, there is no satisfactory explanation.

Perhaps the most helpful answer comes to us from the book of Psalms, where the writer affirms:

> I waited patiently for the Lord,
> He inclined to me and heard my cry.
> He drew me up from the desolate pit,
> Out of the miry bog,
> And set my feet upon a rock,
> Making my steps secure.[6]

8

APPRECIATING HUMOR

"A cheerful heart is a good medicine,
But a downcast spirit dries up the bones."

It is not funny to have arthritis. It would be cruel and insensitive for others to find our situation amusing. But for ourselves, we are confronted with two options—to cry or to laugh. Both are appropriate and natural responses to our condition. For life has both tragic and comic aspects.

A certain amount of crying is therapeutic and relieves the tension and frustration. Yet it is not healthy to become a chronic complainer. Very few people really want to listen to an enumeration of our aches and pains. And little is gained, and much lost, by feeling sorry for ourselves.

LAUGHTER IS HEALING

It is not an easy matter to smile through our tears. Yet there is something redemptive and renewing about laughter. A sense of humor can make a significant difference in dealing with affliction and disability. There is a human tendency for all of us to take ourselves too seriously. Being able to laugh at oneself, to see comedy even in tragedy, can have a healing power. Appreciating humor may be the best medicine. Norman Cousins, in his book <u>Anatomy of an Illness</u>, maintains that laughter was an important part of his capacity to overcome a crippling disease. Here is what he says:

> How scientific was it to believe that laughter—as well as the positive emotions in general—was affecting my body chemistry for the better? If laughter did in fact have a salutary effect on the body's chemistry, it seemed at least theoretically likely that it would enhance the system's ability to fight the inflammation. So we took sedimentation rate readings just before as well as several hours after the laughter episodes. Each time, there was a drop of at least five points. The drop by itself was not substantial, but it held and was cumulative. I was greatly elated by the discovery that there is a physiologic basis for the ancient theory that laughter is good medicine.[7]

To be sure, there are times when it hurts too much to laugh. We try to make some sense out of suffering, but our search seems to lead us nowhere. We find no answers to the question "Why?" We come away unsatisfied, feeling that life is, in many ways a mystery. But life goes on, and the one freedom we have, even in the midst of pain and suffering, is to decide what shall be our attitude toward life's mystery.

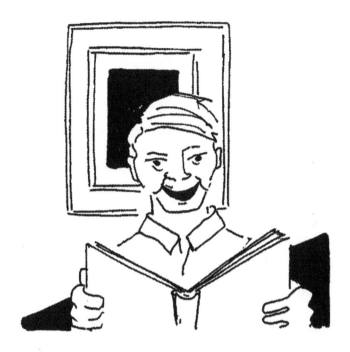

Appreciating Humor

WE SEE WHAT WE LOOK FOR

It has often been said that beauty is in the eye of the beholder. That is to say, we see what we look for. One person sees beauty, another ugliness; one sees hope, another, despair. We can focus either on our possibilities or on our limitations. We can choose whether to see ourselves either as comic or tragic participants in life's unfolding drama.

Sadness and humor are often viewed as contradictory. The truth is that they are complementary, as evidenced by a sad-faced clown. Even in the midst of sadness, humor has a healing quality. It enables us to keep our perspective on life. Humor helps us to see things as they are, and yet have the courage to go on. Sadness can become a burden that weighs heavily upon us; humor makes it possible for us to rise above our situation.

To be sure, there are various kinds of humor. Some humor is sick and mocks others. Healthy humor is never at another person's expense. It is important to know when to laugh, and when to cry, to distinguish between what is funny and what is not.

Developing a sense of humor is something we must do for ourselves. It is a capacity that comes from within. Like medicine, it eases our pains and helps to heal our wounds.

Somewhere I came across this account of the polar Eskimo, written by Gontran de Poncins:

> Here was a people living in the most rigorous climate in the world, in the most depressing surroundings imaginable, haunted by famine in a grey and somber landscape sullen with the absence of life, shivering in their tents in the winter, toiling fifteen hours a day merely in order to get food and stay alive. Huddling and motionless in their igloos through the interminable night, they ought to have been melancholy people, discouraged and despondent. Instead, they were a cheerful people, always laughing, never weary of laughter.[8]

9

EXPRESSING EMOTIONS

"People don't ask for facts in making up their minds. They would rather have one good, soul-satisfying emotion than a dozen facts."

—Robert Keith Leavitt

Emotions are very much a part of our human nature. Our feelings are our natural response to life's situations. Most of us like to think that we are sensible, logical, and rational in our behavior. We believe that our decisions are carefully reasoned out in our minds. It is easy to forget that we are all more influenced by emotion than we are by reason. Our feelings often determine our thinking, whether we are aware of it or not. We are both thinking and feeling creatures.

It is important, therefore, that we give expression to our emotions, rather than suppress them. It is normal for us to experience feelings of fear, anger, guilt, despair, hope, joy, and love. How we deal with our emotions has a great deal to do with our mental, and also physical, health.

EMOTIONS NEITHER RIGHT NOR WRONG

Arthritis, or any other illness, often causes us to feel angry about our affliction, fearful of the future, guilty, about our past mistakes, and despairing about our situation. It is essential, therefore, to find appropriate ways in which to express these emotions.

It is not a question of whether it is right or wrong to feel as we do. The honest thing is to acknowledge that we do feel the way we do and then proceed to deal constructively with this feeling. It is no help at all, and can be harmful, for someone to tell us "You should not feel the way you do."

To deny our genuine emotions is to keep them inside ourselves where they can affect our sense of well-being. There is a great deal of dishonesty and deceit regarding emotions. We sometimes act brave to conceal our fear; we smile to cover up our anger; we boast about our exploits when we really feel guilty; we seek all kinds of escape from our despair. All these are inappropriate responses to genuine emotions. There is no need to feel ashamed for feeling as we do.

POSITIVE AND NEGATIVE

Emotions are of two kinds—positive and negative. Positive emotions are joy, hope, and love. Negative emotions are fear, anger, guilt, and despair. It seems to be true that we must try to work through our negative feelings before we can begin to experience our positive feelings. That is why this book follows the pattern of discussing negative factors before going on to affirm the positive ones. All of us want to find happiness and affection and contentment, but our negative attitudes stand in the way, like roadblocks barring our travel along the road to fulfillment. The roadblocks must be removed before we can reach our intended destination.

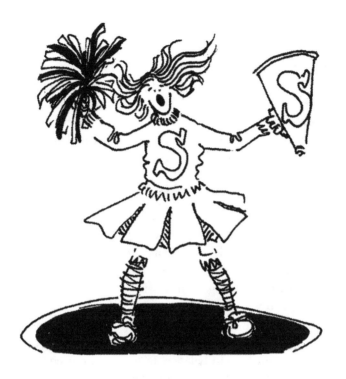

Expressing Emotions

Those of us who seek to conceal our deeper feelings sometimes envy the person who can "let it all hang out." We think how good it must feel to be able to let our emotions explode, to "blow our top." But the person who acts out his or her highly-charged emotions often admits privately that there is a heavy burden of guilt that follows after having overtly demonstrated negative emotions. One says and does things which, having been said and done, cannot be changed or erased.

There are times when it is not possible, under the circumstances, to openly express our feelings. The risk of displaying our anger toward our employer may be too threatening. All too often, a wife and children become the innocent victims of a hostility that is safer to express at home than at work.

KEEPING OUR EMOTIONAL BALANCE

How, then, can we express emotions constructively, rather than destructively? One of the ways in which we can work through emotions that cannot be expressed elsewhere is to confide in a professional counselor, or even with an understanding friend who is a good listener. By what is called "transference" we can dispose of our pent-up feelings with a safe listener, one who will not betray our confidence and who will not take personally what we say. Usually there is a sense of relief when we have "dumped" our anger or guilt on someone who can be an understanding listener and who will still accept us in spite of how we feel.

The goal is to keep our lives in balance, to maintain our equilibrium. Being a healthy, whole person necessitates balancing our thoughts, feelings, and behavior. Letting our emotions run wild, or denying that we have emotions, are both extremes to be avoided. Controlling our emotions is not the same as refusing to admit our feelings. Perhaps there is always a healthy tension between how we think and how we feel that determines our attitudes and actions.

10

FACING REALITY

"Do what you can, with what you have, where you are."

—Theodore Roosevelt

"Say it isn't so! Tell me this isn't really happening to me!" It is deeply disturbing to have our customary way of life abruptly interrupted by some unexpected problem. Our hope is that it is some temporary, passing inconvenience. Surely tomorrow will be better. We simply do not want to believe that some misfortune, some illness, some disability has overtaken us.

Our first reaction to arthritis, then, is denial. We prefer to pretend that it isn't really so. We refuse to admit it to others, and especially to ourselves. Confronted with the choice of fight or flight, we try to run away from our situation, to escape from reality.

THE GRIEF PROCESS

Being told that we have a chronic disease like arthritis is a grief experience, like any other sad and unhappy life event. According to Dr. Elisabeth Kubler-Ross, there are several stages through which grieving persons usually pass. These stages are denial, anger, bargaining, depression, and acceptance.[9] A whole emotional process is involved before we are ready to face reality. The full impact of any misfortune is too great for us to deal with at one time. Step by step, we are gradually, though painfully, able to absorb and assimilate the shock.

Grief must be expressed; feelings need to surface. We may choose to express grief privately, rather than publicly. But we must do our "grief work" or grief will take a heavy toll upon our mental and physical well-being. It requires courage to move from the realm of fantasy and make-believe to the world of reality. Good mental health necessitates facing reality. The alternative is mental illness, which is characterized by being out of touch with the real world.

THE CHOICE BEFORE US

What are you going to do about your arthritis? Are you going to give up in despair? Are you going to cling to false hopes that it will disappear? Are you going to spend your time and money searching for a miracle cure? The time comes for an honest, soul-searching, self-examination. What is reality for you? You need to develop realistic expectations for yourself.

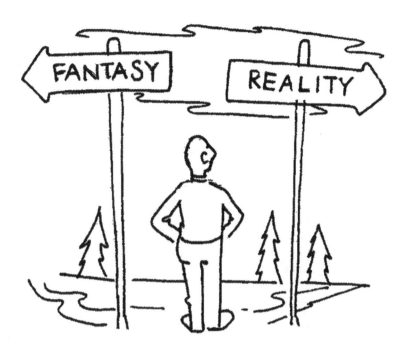

Facing Reality

Many people, in wellness or illness, have unrealistic expectations for themselves and for others. They set impossible goals, become perfectionists, and are constantly unhappy in an imperfect world. But especially for anyone who suffers from arthritis, as well as other disabling diseases, it is essential to set realistic goals that are possible for you to achieve. Instead of trying to accomplish too many things, and feeling frustrated, establish achievable goals for that morning or afternoon, and feel the satisfaction of having completed what you set out to do.

In dealing with arthritis, it is important to distinguish between realistic expectations and false hopes. On the positive side, doctors now have available a wide-ranging variety of arthritic medications. If one kind does not help, your doctor will try another. All medications should be taken under close supervision. Sometimes it is necessary to increase or decrease the dosage, according to your own needs. Some of these prescribed medications have side-effects, which you should ask your doctor to discuss before undertaking any program of medication.

New drugs are continually being developed. However, before these are made available, they must be thoroughly tested in order to determine possible harmful side-effects. What is encouraging is that much progress is being made in the treatment of arthritis in its various forms.

Most people can control their arthritis with proper medication, rest, exercise, and joint activity. However, various surgical procedures have been developed for those where joint damage has occurred. Surgery is now performed for various joints—hand and wrist, hip, elbow, knee, ankle. Most successful has been hip replacements, although there is now sufficient experience with knee replacement to justify consideration of this possibility. Before any surgery is undertaken, however, careful and thoughtful attention must be given to the risks involved and the prognosis for improvement. A rheumatologist should evaluate your total situation before any specific procedures are undertaken. He will, if so indicated, recommend specialists who perform particular kinds of joint surgery. Here, also, much progress has taken place, partly as the result of athletic injuries.

In sharp contrast to proven medical procedures are an abundance of false promises held out by unproven remedies. Included among these are drugs, diets, plants and herbs, venoms, devices, lotions and ointments, and miscellaneous remedies. Although extravagant claims are made for these so-called "cures," none of them have been subjected to scientifically designed trials. Often well-meaning friends or relatives suggest such methods, which may be either expensive or border on the ridiculous.

In the book, Understanding Arthritis, edited by the Arthritis Foundation, the following ways are given for recognizing unproven remedies:

1. A cure is offered.

2. The remedy is described as a "secret" formula.

3. Testimonials are offered as "proof."

4. The remedy is described in sensational tabloids.

5. Quick, simple relief of pain is promised.

6. The treatment promises cleansing of body "toxins."

7. Drugs and surgery are condemned.

8. No reliable evidence or scientific proof is offered.

9. A special diet or nutrition program is promoted.

10. The medical profession is accused of conspiracy.[10]

It should be emphasized that each person's situation is different. Treatment programs need to be individualized, and there is no "miracle cure" that can solve our health problems. Since each of us is a unique human being, it is neither wise nor healthy to compare ourselves to others or to experiment with the methods they use to deal with their arthritis. Instead of pursuing false hopes, it is the better part of wisdom to face reality and to rely on tried and tested methods of treatment.

11

RE-ASSESSING VALUES

"Values do not drive a man; they do not push him, but rather pull him."

—Viktor Frankl

"How much is it worth?" is a more important question than "How much does it cost?" If something is of value to us, we are willing to pay any price, make any sacrifice, to possess it. For the pearl of great price, we are willing to surrender all our pearls of lesser value. What is of worth to one person may be worthless to another. Someone once suggested that life is like a display window, in which some mischievous person has re-arranged the price tags, placing a high price tag on cheap things, and a lower cost on more precious things.

Situations change, and our values change. What mattered most when we were young is not the same as what is most important to us in later years. James Russell Lowell wrote that "new occasions teach new duties."

A NEW BALL GAME

Illness or disability confronts us with a new situation which causes us to re-assess our values. The inability to engage in activities we once did brings us face to face with both our limitations and our possibilities. It is a new ball game, and new rules need to be formulated.

Hospitalization and convalescence are often occasions for serious reflection on our customary lifestyle. In good health, we waste a great deal of time and energy in spinning our wheels. When fatigue, exhaustion, stiffness, or pain are our frequent companions, we are confronted with the necessity to conserve our resources. The person who has difficulty in walking learns to use the telephone and "let his fingers do the walking." The person who finds writing legibly a problem may resort to using an electric computer or a micro-cassette recorder.

Whether we realize it or not, our values shape our actions. We become what we believe. The behavior of others, or even ourselves, would not perplex us so much if we understood the motives and values which prompt those actions. The relentless pursuit of a goal often results in the end justifying the means.

Often our values are influenced by our society or those with whom we associate. It is a great concern that so many place material values above spiritual values. The Bible tells us that "a man's life does not consist in the abundance of his possessions."(Luke 12:15)

THE ESSENTIAL VALUE

Illness confronts us with the reality that there are things that money cannot buy, among them good health. Dealing with disease or disability calls upon one's inner, spiritual resources. When the flesh is weak, the spirit needs to be strong.

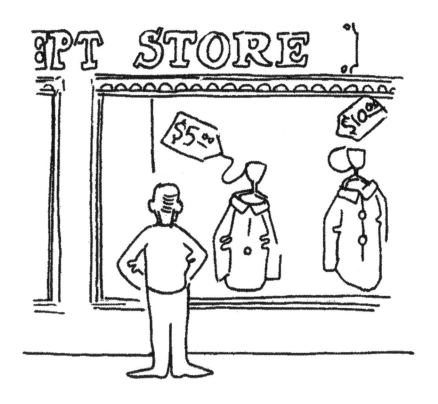

Re-assessing Values

The changed circumstances brought about by severe arthritis necessitate our adapting to change and reorganizing our value system. This enforced confrontation can bring a peace of mind that enables us to accept our situation and find greater meaning in our existence. Perhaps this is a blessing that comes from suffering.

As some doors close, others open for us. Since the essential value is life itself, we let go of the past and reach out to the future. What we have left is more vital than what we have lost.

The example of others can greatly benefit us in making our own value judgments. There are always those persons whom we greatly admire for the manner in which they bear adversity. Seeking to emulate others can strengthen us in our own resolve to find the strength and courage that we need for the living of our days. Physical limitations need not keep us from maintaining, to the best of our ability, the moral and ethical values that we cherish.

Dr. Paul Tournier, the famous Swiss psychologist, tells of this incident:

> In the street one day I met a former patient whose serious illness caused me a lot of worry at the time. He is obviously pleased to meet me again, and remarks in a jocular tone that is not meant to hide his seriousness, "Oh, doctor, you know that I have very happy memories of that time. It was tough, all right, but looking back, it seems to me that it was one of the most fruitful periods of my life. I learned more in those few months of my illness than in twenty years of good health.[11]

12

PLANNING AHEAD

"It is important to plan in order not to fall back-first into the future."

—Paul Valery

One of the problems related to arthritis is that one never knows when there may be a flare-up. Such incidents can occur at the most inconvenient times, incapacitating one for days at a time. Unwelcome as flare-ups are, they are part of the reality of being afflicted with arthritis.

Can flare-ups be avoided? Yes! The secret lies in learning to plan ahead, to pace yourself. Try to avoid over-exertion, exhaustion, and stressful situations. This means developing the discipline to plan ahead. Limiting responsibilities and working in advance are necessary requisites for living with arthritis.

EXPECT THE UNEXPECTED

Procrastination, putting things off, may be an option for many people, but it is not a real possibility for arthritics. Waiting until the last minute may result in being unprepared. It is essential to expect the unexpected and allow for it by pacing oneself.

When expecting to have a busy evening, adequate rest during the day is the wise thing. When facing a heavy schedule, try to avoid letting responsibilities pile up. We all have limits to our endurance, and this is especially true of arthritics. Planning ahead is an essential way to avoid flare-ups.

Most people waste a great deal of time and energy. Because they are in relatively good health, they do not find it necessary to organize their time or conserve their energy.

If you have arthritis, you may no longer be able to do all the things that other people do, or all the things that you formerly did. This may be a loss, but it may also be a gain. You will, of necessity, choose those activities that are most meaningful and important to you. You may, for example, use the telephone to call friends instead of visiting them; you may place orders and pay bills by mail, instead of running around to stores; if your walking is impaired, as mine is, you will learn ways to get jobs done with the minimum of effort. Life, in some ways, becomes simpler, less frantic.

LEARN TO SAY "NO"

All of us are, at times, overwhelmed by the multiplicity of things needing to be done. A sense of inadequacy overpowers us, and we feel completely ineffective. But most of us are capable of doing only one thing at a time. We discover that by making a beginning, taking one step at a time, we are able to succeed in meeting our obligations.

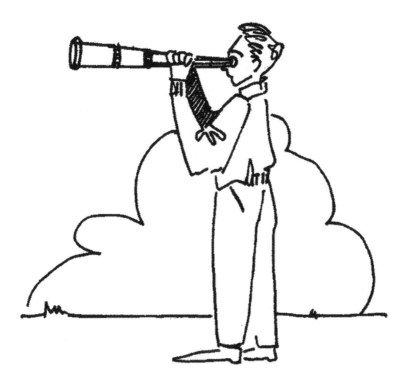

Planning Ahead

Each day, prepare a checklist of duties needing to be performed. Arrange your list in order of importance, first things first. Try to have a manageable list, rather than attempting to do too many things in one day. Guard against overloading yourself.

One of the lessons many people never learn is how to say "No!" Realizing your limitations requires having the good judgment to refuse those tasks that cause uptightness and tension, unless your job description leaves no alternative. To some extent—depending upon your type of employment—each person has the capacity to select and organize his or her own activities, particularly leisure pastimes.

Planning ahead and pacing ourselves is a way of learning to live with arthritis. By anticipating the unexpected it is possible to live a productive and meaningful life.

13

SETTING PRIORITIES

"It is not enough to be busy.
The question is: What are we busy about?"

—Henry David Thoreau

Recovering from a hip fracture, I spent most of the summer sitting on the front porch of our house, carrying on only minimal responsibilities. Suddenly, I had been interrupted in the midst of a busy and active life. Hopping around on one foot for three months isn't the best way to get things done. My friends nick-named me "Hopalong." My son built a long ramp with siderails so I could get up and down the front steps. Instead of my rushing around in the world, I was now in the position of waiting for the world to come to my doorstep.

Sitting there, hour after hour, I had time to do a great deal of thinking. No longer able to do all the things I was accustomed to doing, I pondered over those things which were most urgent. Having heard a great deal about setting priorities, I now found that I needed to establish some priorities of my own. Knowing that I could not do everything, I rejected the notion of doing nothing, and deter-mined that there were still some things I could do. Fortunately, my job was of such a nature that I could make my own decisions about ranking the relative importance of different parts of my job description.

FIRST THINGS FIRST

If we fail to organize our activities, we are likely to waste a great deal of time and energy. If we are temporarily slowed down, we have an opportunity to observe how hyperactive many people are. There appears to be a need, on the part of most of us, to fill up as many as possible of the empty moments of our lives. We speak with a mixture of pride and complaint about how busy we are. There is an almost frantic air about our human activity, as though being busy somehow justi-fies our existence. We seldom take time to organize our lives until necessity deter-mines the need for us.

What merits highest priority in your life? What is most important to you? Unfortunately, for some it is no longer possible, when faced with illness or injury, to continue their present employment. For some people who suffer from arthri-tis, joint deformity, muscle deconditioning, morning stiffness, or lack of energy, it may be necessary to seek some new form of employment. Occupational reha-bilitation, for some, may be the highest priority.

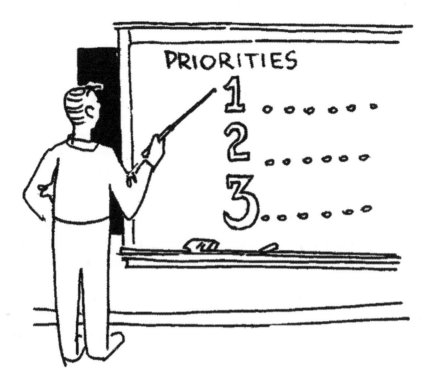

Setting Priorities

MAKING CHANGES

In my own case, even with decreased mobility, I was able to carry on many of the most important parts of my work. It was necessary to find alternative ways of dealing with other responsibilities. Colleagues took over the, functions that I could no longer perform. I learned how to use the telephone more frequently, ordered supplies from catalogues, and sent letters to people I was unable to visit. Being slowed down, I learned how to set priorities, became better organized, and functioned more efficiently. Amazingly, I found this to be more satisfying—as well as more relaxing—than waiting until the last minute to resort to burning the midnight oil. Instead of feeling under pressure, it actually lifted my spirits to be able to carry on in spite of my limitations.

It is regrettable that developing priorities may mean giving up some of the activities one enjoys most. More is involved than merely eliminating the tasks which one finds tedious and tiresome. Having temporary or permanent disabilities requires a careful evaluation of what one is able to do and what most needs to be done.

Instead of yielding to despair and hopelessness because of unwelcome limitations, the willingness to set priorities indicates that we are making an honest attempt to carry on, under very altered circumstances, doing what we can, with what we have, where we are.

14

MAINTAINING INDEPENDENCE

"Independence is the freedom to survey all of the available alternatives in a given situation and then use this collected information to make a conscious choice."

—A. Cappaert

Rugged individualism is greatly admired, but it is an outdated concept in our complex, modern world. It was a quality that characterized the pioneer spirit in early America, but increasingly we have become less independent, and more interdependent, in a shrinking world. The philosophy of "every man for himself" is no longer possible in our global village. We all need each other.

Dependency is an unpopular idea, implying weakness and inadequacy. It seems especially true that as arthritics we want to do things for ourselves, instead of having others do them for us. This is probably a healthy attitude, one which enables us to maintain our dignity and self-respect. However, the reality is that we are no longer able to do everything for ourselves. Mutual dependency is a fact of life.

THE DEPENDENT-INDEPENDENT ISSUE

One of the insights, therefore, that arthritics need to gain is how to be dependent, to a lesser or greater degree, upon others. Particularly if we are fortunate enough to live with caring family members, we need to learn how to accept help graciously. When struggling with buttons, shoelaces, or bottle caps, why is it so difficult for us to accept help?

To be sure, we want to maintain our independence as much as possible. Disabled people have been known to tyrannize their families with their affliction, demanding immediate attention. Basically, it is better to do things for ourselves, rather than to have others do them for us. But somehow we need to face up to the truth that others want to be of help, that this is a way of their sharing our suffering, and that we do, at times, need assistance.

There will likely always be a certain tension about the dependency-independency issue. But the effects of arthritis make it necessary for us to realize that we are, at least partially, dependent upon others. In this respect, we are not so different from everyone else. We are, none of us, isolated individuals, each living in a separate, little world. We are social beings, sharing life's experiences, both of joy and sorrow, health and sickness, prosperity and adversity. Being of help to one another enriches the life of both the one giving and the one receiving. Admitting our dependence is not a sign of weakness. It may well be a sign of humility and strength.

In her study entitled <u>Physical Disability: A Psychosocial Approach</u>, Beatrice Wright has this to say:

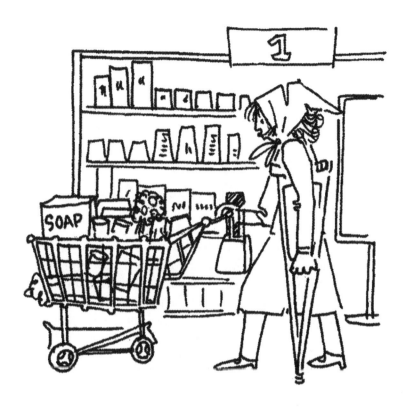

Maintaining Independence

Just as people may be excessively dependent on others, they may also be excessively independent of others. In both instances the person is denying the self and others certain values. Excessive dependency denies the obvious value of ability to do for oneself and accomplish certain goals. Excessive independence denies the less accepted value of emotional sharing. It also constricts one's range of accomplishment by negating the desirability of relying on others and delegating responsibility. Being goaded by independence, the person may insist on doing for himself only to be depleted of energy and emotional resources that might have been spent more usefully.[12]

We do not want others to be insensitive or indifferent to our suffering. Inwardly we long for empathy and understanding from those we encounter. Yet we often fail to see life from the perspective of those who sincerely want to be helpful. That is their way of showing that they care. Without surrendering our self-esteem, we can learn to accept help and not feel threatened or obligated.

Receiving help should not be a one-way street. There are also ways in which we, in spite of our limitations, can also give help. Perhaps the key to the dependency-independency tension hinges upon the word "necessary" assistance. Otherwise, we prefer to do things for ourselves. In summary, we need to learn how and when to be appropriately dependent upon others, just as we need to learn when to be independent.

15

TAKING RESPONSIBILITY

"Life ultimately means taking the responsibility to find the right answer to its problems and to fulfill the tasks which it constantly sets for each individual."

—Viktor Frankl

A young woman was applying for a job. During the interview, she was asked the question: "Are you responsible?" Her reply was: "Oh, yes. Where I worked before, whenever anything went wrong, they said I was responsible."

For good or bad, you are the person who is responsible for your health care. Our natural inclination is to place the burden of responsibility on our doctor. We expect him or her to find out what is our problem, and to do something about it. It is appropriate that we turn to the medical profession for diagnosis and treatment, and this is especially true with the various forms of arthritis. It is a serious mistake to rely on over-the-counter remedies that promise relief from arthritis pain. Too many people have waited too long before consulting a family physician or rheumatologist. Millions of dollars are spent each year by people who are seeking relief from pain and discomfort. Probably no group of sufferers is more victimized than arthritics. For a disease that presently has no known cure, it is incredible to consider the number of miracle cures and quack formulas that are available.

A TEAM EFFORT

In view of the chronic, up and down, nature of arthritis, it is the patient who must take the responsibility for carrying out a treatment program. If you do not take charge and follow your individualized treatment program, no one else will. Dealing with arthritis is a team effort, involving doctors, therapists, and other health professionals, but you yourself must faithfully carry out the treatment program, even during the times when you are free from flare-ups or when your arthritis is in remission.

No one can live with arthritis without some organized plan, including medication, exercise, and rest. Applying such a program cannot be sporadic, carried out only during flare-ups and neglected during remissions, but instead must be consistently followed.

There is a real temptation to discontinue exercise, medications, and other treatment during trouble-free periods. I have personally found it very difficult to carry out a regular exercise program. It is relatively easy to have a physical therapist guide you through an exercise program in a hospital. At home, working alone, is another story. The solution probably lies in having a family member or a close friend to work with you, if that is possible. If you must work alone, it requires great self-discipline. However, once regular times are established, like any other habit, exercise becomes a part of your daily routine.

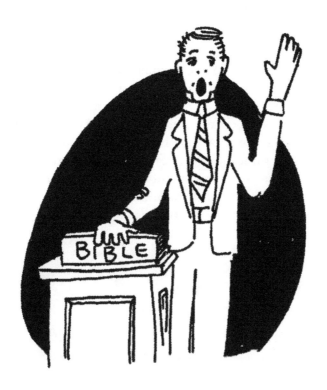

Taking Responsibility

TOO MUCH OR TOO LITTLE

Whether you are feeling good or bad, prescribed medications must be taken regularly, as directed. Do not increase or decrease the dosage without the permission of your physician. Above all, do not try someone else's medications. Aspirin, the old standby for arthritis, is easily available, but in order to be effective, your doctor needs to determine your maximum tolerable dosage. Laboratory tests are also essential at regular intervals to determine the effects of various medications.

Although you must take responsibility for following your treatment program, a doctor, preferably a rheumatologist, needs to work out an individualized treatment plan according to your particular situation. Too much exercise, too much rest, or too much medication can do as much harm as good. The bottom line is that, under your doctor's supervision, you need to take charge—you are responsible.

16

DEVELOPING EMPATHY

"Empathy is a process whereby one person perceives accurately another person's feelings and the meaning of those feelings and then communicates with sensitivity this understanding to the other person."

—Kenneth Bullmer

Someone has said that we should care for others as though we were the others. Often we become so preoccupied with our own problems that we are indifferent to what others may be experiencing. It is difficult for us to identify with others unless we ourselves have had a similar experience.

Pain and discomfort can easily make us self-centered. We are inclined to focus upon our own aches and pains and mistakenly conclude that all is well with others. There is always the temptation to feel sorry for ourselves, which results in a descending spiral of frustration and despair.

WAYS OF RESPONDING

It is safe to assume that virtually everyone, at some time, has some burden to bear. Although not everyone, fortunately, is faced with a chronic condition like arthritis, many people are confronted with some kind of physical or emotional crisis in their personal or family life.

Our own suffering can open our eyes to the difficulties of others around us. It is possible for us to feel a greater sensitivity for what others may be enduring. Any disability of our own can give us greater empathy toward the problems and infirmities of others.

There is much pathos, or sadness, in life. We respond to the unfortunate elements of life either with apathy, sympathy, or empathy. Many people are completely unmoved, apathetic, toward the adversities of others. Some respond emotionally, with tears of sympathy. But we need to strive for empathy, that is, entering into, sharing in, what others are experiencing.

The Native Americans have a saying that one must walk for a mile in the other brave's moccasins. Afflictions have the possibility of isolating us in a solitary world, or they can bring us closer to one another as we share one another's burdens. Any load becomes lighter when someone helps us to carry it.

HOW CAN I HELP?

How does one show empathy? To begin, draw upon your own experiences. What actions of others were helpful to you? What were some things that people might have done, but did not do, that would have been meaningful to you?

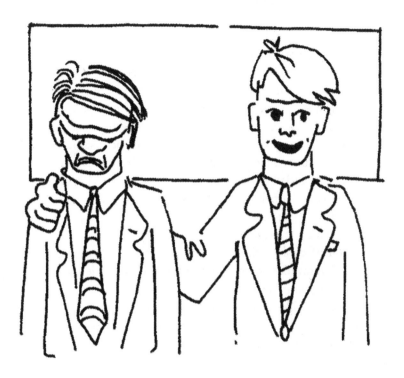

Developing Empathy

To a large extent, the ways in which you choose to show that you care depends upon your own imagination and ability. Few actions mean more than a personal visit. Although visiting has largely gone out of style, most of us welcome someone stopping by just to be together. It is puzzling that many people who visit patients in a hospital forget that sometimes convalescence is an even more tedious period of time. Several short visits are better than one long one.

Because of distance or your own inability to get about, you may decide to send a card, or preferably, to write a note of encouragement. An occasional telephone call will let someone know that you are thinking of the person. Sometimes a telephone call is even more convenient than having someone stop by for a visit. If the person has a tape recorder, and enjoys music, a cassette of his or her favorite kind of music is a pleasant surprise. With the increasing availability of talking books, this makes a welcome gift to a convalescent or homebound person.

If you have a garden, a few flowers can brighten someone's day. If you are able to bake, a batch of cookies shows a personal touch. Much depends upon your own ability and resourcefulness, but the best guideline is what you might like someone to do for you in a similar situation.

We are all more alike than we are different. Just as we ourselves yearn for understanding, so others also have the same longing. Perhaps much of the meaning of life is found in trying to make life better for one another.

17

FINDING FAITH

Man cannot live without faith, because the prime requisite in life's adventure is courage, and the sustenance of courage is faith. "

—Harry Emerson Fosdick

The shield has been the traditional symbol for faith. Confronted with any crisis, we need something to protect ourselves. Some people may ask: "Does it matter what you believe?" What we believe makes all the difference in the world, for, in a real sense, we become what we believe. Take away our beliefs, remove the shield of faith, and we are defenseless against life's obstacles.

We need to believe in someone or something beyond ourselves. There is power inherent in the universe, and we must plug into that source of power. Electricity is a powerful force, but unless we make contact, it is useless. The real vitality of life resides, not in ourselves, but outside us and beyond us. My own personal experience is that what overcomes adversity is faith in God, in some supreme being, who created us, who sustains us throughout our lives.

WHERE IS OUR HOPE?

The Bible tells us that God's strength is made perfect in our weakness. Our human inadequacies can lead to despair unless we can find sufficiency beyond our own limitations.

St. Paul, who himself suffered from a physical disability, wrote out of his own experience that "suffering produces endurance, and endurance produces character, and character produces hope, and hope does not disappoint us." (Romans 5:3) This same process that St. Paul described can be realized in our lives as well. Our true hope lies, not in relentlessly pursuing some miracle cure, but rather in accepting our disability and trusting that God will give us the strength to endure. "Though our outer nature is wasting away, our inner nature is being renewed every day." (2 Corinthians 4:16)

The popular religion of our time is humanism, which places all its faith in what man and woman can do. My own conviction is that this is a deception. By ourselves alone, we simply are not adequate to the tragedies of life. Just as we must develop relationships with other persons in order to survive, so we must also develop a relationship with the one who created us and endowed us with the gift of life. We are not just physical bodies that often hurt; we are also spiritual beings, endowed with a spirit that can triumph over affliction. This body of ours is a house in which a spirit dwells. How we nurture that spirit within us is just as important as now we nourish our bodies.

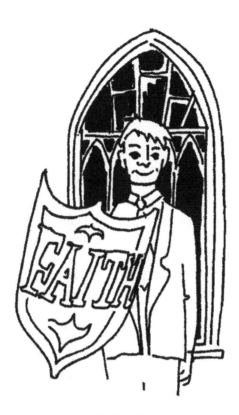

Finding Faith

THE HEALING POWER OF FAITH

There are those who claim to be "faith healers," but whether they acknowledge it or not, healing power comes from God. There is a healing power within the human body, a natural capacity to restore health. But sometimes disease interrupts this healing process. For some of us, the answer to our illness lies, not in physical healing, but in spiritual healing. It may not be possible for us to have our bodies cured of arthritis, but our healing may be expressed through a spirit that enables us to endure.

In his book, <u>The Dynamics of Faith</u>, Paul Tillich writes:

> The healing power of faith is related to the whole personality, independent of any special disease of body or mind, and effective positively or negatively in every moment of one's life. It precedes, accompanies, and follows all other activities of healing … Medical activities, including mental healing, cannot produce a reintegration of the personality as a whole. Only faith can do that.[13]

We face our situation being either faithless or faithful. We cannot hope to find meaning in our suffering unless we have faith in ourselves and others. Above all, we need to find faith in a power beyond ourselves, which we call God. "By ourselves we can do nothing, but with God all things are possible." (Matthew 19:26) "Lord, I believe; help my unbelief." (Mark 9:24)

The following lines, entitled "Unanswered Prayer," were found on the body of an unknown Confederate soldier:

> I asked God for strength, that I might achieve,
> I was made weak, that I might learn humbly to obey.
> I asked for health, that I might do greater things,
> I was given infirmity, that I might do better things.
> I asked for riches, that I might be happy,
> I was given poverty, that I might be wise.
> I asked for power, that I might have the praise of men,
> I was given weakness, that I might feel the need of God.
> I asked for all things, that I might enjoy life,
> I was given life, that I might enjoy all things.
> I got nothing that I asked for—but everything I had hoped for.

Almost despite myself, my unspoken prayers are answered.
I am among all people most richly blessed.[14]

18

STRENGTHENING SELF-ESTEEM

"Oftentimes nothing profits more than self-esteem, Grounded in what is just and right."

—John Milton

We live in a time when great emphasis is placed on health and fitness. People of all ages are walking more, running more, and exercising more. Much of this is beneficial and contributes to a sense of well-being. However, it can have an adverse effect upon those of us who suffer from arthritis or other disabilities. Since we cannot participate fully in physical fitness programs, except to a limited degree, we are inclined to feel a sense of inadequacy. If good health contributes to a person's sense of self-esteem, then poor health can result in a loss of self-esteem. Our limitations can cause us to feel inferior to others.

ADOPT A POSITIVE ATTITUDE

A major task of learning to live with arthritis is that of maintaining and strengthening our self-esteem. Instead of losing confidence in ourselves, we need to adopt a positive attitude toward our situation. How we perceive ourselves is an important factor in how others perceive us. If we see ourselves as sick and crippled, others will very likely treat us accordingly. However, if we maintain, as much as possible, our self-confidence and self-worth, others will be guided by that evaluation.

In his book, <u>Living With Your Arthritis</u>, Dr. Alan Rosenberg states:

> A common problem among people with a chronic illness is loss of self-esteem. Self-esteem is a term meaning self-respect or satisfaction with oneself. Illness often forces us to turn inward, and as a result we may dwell upon our problems excessively. Especially if our mobility is impaired, we feel that we can do very little about even small problems and so we lose our incentive to try to come to grips with our illness. We may despair at accomplishing even necessary daily living tasks. Such despair leads to depression and loss of self-esteem. [15]

What reason is there to think less of ourselves after the onset of an illness than we did before? Are we not the same persons? Is our sense of well-being the result of what we can do, or of who we are? Isn't it more basic to be than to do? It is just possible that, because our affliction has caused us to re-assess our values, we might conceivably be more mature, productive persons than before.

MIND OVER BODY

Good mental health need not necessarily be destroyed by poor physical health. One of the amazing qualities of our human nature is the capacity to determine what kind of thoughts and attitudes we will have. It is, after all, our minds that give instructions to our bodies. Since this is true, it is our mental outlook that can determine how we view our illness.

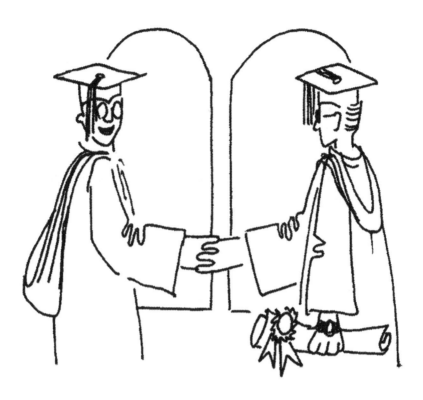

Strengthening Self-esteem

We are spiritual, as well as physical, beings. It is the human spirit that has triumphed over all manner of adversity. Three hundred years ago, Robert Burton observed:

> Deformities and imperfections of our bodies, as lameness, crookedness, deafness, blindness, be they innate or accidental, torture many men; yet this may comfort them that those imperfections of the body do not a whit blemish the soul, or hinder the operations of it, but rather help and much increase it.[16]

It is possible, then, believe it or not, for a disabled person to have a healthier outlook on life than an able-bodied person may have. Good health is so much taken for granted that those in poor physical health may sometimes develop a healthier perspective on life than the physically fit.

Each of us has worth and value as a person. In order to overcome our arthritis, we need to strengthen our sense of self-esteem. You are no less a person now than you were before.

19

SHARING PROBLEMS

"The fellowship of those who bear the mark of pain—who are the members of this fellowship? Those who have learned by experience what physical and bodily anguish mean, belong together all the world over: they are united by a secret bond. One and all, they know the horrors of suffering to which man can be exposed, and one and all, they know the longing to be free from pain."

—Albert Schweitzer

Perhaps you have heard the comment that "true happiness lies in sharing with others." The original intent was very likely a reference to sharing possessions, but it might also apply to sharing problems and concerns. Living with arthritis can be an unhappy burden, however, sharing our problems with others who are similarly afflicted lightens the load. Instead of keeping our misery inside ourselves, we can find in fellow-sufferers, as well as in caring family members and friends, listening ears and helping hands. For those who live with arthritics do share in the pain and discomfort. They, too, are frustrated when there is nothing that can be done about our situation. A wife or husband may wish there were some magic words that could be spoken to alleviate our suffering.

SUPPORT GROUPS

Without becoming a chronic complainer, you need to develop openness to discussing your disease. You will be able to distinguish between those persons who are just being polite and those who are genuinely interested in listening. Often honesty and frankness on your part will enable others to share your problems.

This sharing of concerns is particularly valuable with others who may also be troubled with arthritis. There is a kind of fellowship of suffering among persons sharing the same, or similar, problems. This mutual need has resulted in the formation of support groups. It is helpful, at times, to be in the company of a group that shares our limitations.

Alcoholics Anonymous is a shining example of people who share the same problem and thereby become mutually supportive. You might think that such sharing would have a negative effect, feeling sorry for each other. However, in actuality, the results are very positive. Group members learn from each other how to cope with their problem in ways that they might not have discovered for themselves.

A simple illustration will serve to show the value of group sharing. If you have a dollar, and I have a dollar, and you give me your dollar, and I give you my dollar, each of us still has just one dollar. However, if you have an idea, and I have an idea, and you give me your idea, and I give you my idea, each of us then has two ideas.

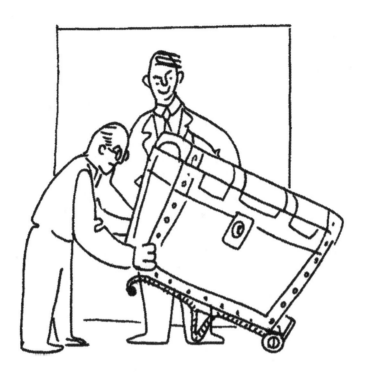

Sharing Problems

MEMBERS OF A TEAM

We find inspiration and encouragement in seeing how others deal with their problems. We go away feeling that we are not the only ones in the world grappling daily with a difficult situation. We can learn, even from one another's mistakes. Such mutual support groups for arthritics now exist in many communities. Your local Arthritis Foundation chapter can put you in touch with existing groups or give you direction in forming one.

To overcome the feeling of isolation, it also helps to remember that you are a member of a team, composed of your doctor, other health professionals, family members, and friends. It is not enough, however, to depend on your doctor to solve your problems, or to lean on family members, expecting them to anticipate your needs. You yourself must take responsibility for dealing with your health problems, and the other team members can advise and assist you in your efforts. You may, depending upon your situation, need a visiting nurse, a physical therapist, a counselor, or some other helping person. But none of these can do for you what you can only do for yourself—take the responsibility for your problems.

There appear to be two groups of people in the world—those who care, and those who do not care. Sometimes you may think that no one cares what happens to you, but that simply is not true. You cannot just sit and wait for people to reach out to you; you must also reach out to others. If you can develop a wholesome, positive attitude toward your problems, there are many people who will care, and who will share.

20

OVERCOMING ARTHRITIS

"When the morning's freshness has been replaced by the weariness of midday, and the muscles quiver under the strain, the climb seems endless, and, suddenly, nothing will go quite as you wish—it is then that you must not stop."

—Dag Hammerskjold

One of the most remarkable qualities that we possess is the capacity to adapt to new situations. Life is dynamic, not static, and changes are continually taking place within us and around us. Change may be either good or bad, but our chances for survival depend largely upon how well we adjust to change. There is some evidence that arthritics tend to be rigid personalities, but in order to overcome arthritis, we must learn to develop flexibility.

Confronted with any crisis, two possible options immediately present themselves—flight or fight. Our first impulse is to run away, to escape from an unpleasant situation. Faced with the reality of arthritis, some individuals never stop running, endlessly pursuing some miracle cure. Arthritics are the most victimized of all sufferers. Exploiting our pain is a profitable business. Quackery abounds, and because of our discomfort, we are gullible customers.

FRIEND OR ENEMY?

If flight is not the answer, is it possible for us to fight against our condition? In a very true sense, we need to be fighters, refusing to give up, always ready to fight one more round. Instead of surrendering, we must resist. Instead of sinking, we need to swim. Yet, in another sense, what determines defeat or victory is not struggle, but acceptance. Having experienced the stages of denial, anger, frustration, and depression, the hope is that we can finally come to terms with the reality of our situation, which means accepting things as they are.

Abraham Lincoln once said: "The best way to get rid of an enemy is to make a friend out of him." Can arthritis possibly be seen as a friend, rather than an enemy? To be sure, it is an unwelcome guest in our bodies, yet, an intruder that has moved in either temporarily or permanently.

Our peace of mind depends upon how well we adjust to living in the same body with arthritis, although we would prefer to kick the rascal out. In miniature, our personal problems are similar to the larger problem of hostile nations with differing ideologies finding ways for co-existing in one world. We may not like our neighbors, but instead of destroying each other, we continue the quest for peace on earth. Overcoming arthritis is not ultimately a matter of getting rid of it—although we wish we could do that—but, more realistically, of learning to live with it.

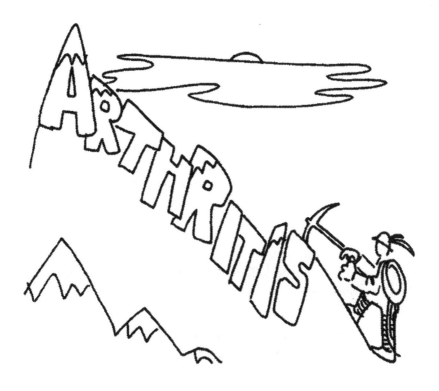

Overcoming Arthritis

ONE DAY AT A TIME

The bottom line in overcoming arthritis is motivation. All the best efforts of doctors, health team members, and family are insufficient unless you, the arthritic, have the desire and determination to work through your situation. This is no easy task, but is there really any other choice? Who else, but you, can take the initiative and responsibility for what needs to be done?

We are gifted with the freedom to choose what kind of thoughts and attitudes will guide our behavior. "The thought is father of the deed." We can, on the one hand, resent our limitations, yield to frustration, give in to depression, lose our patience. On the other hand, we can choose to make the best of a bad situation, accept our limitations, master our depression, cultivate patience. The choice lies with us.

Fortunately, we live only one day at a time. It is too much to confront at one moment all the days, or months, or years, that lie ahead. What matters most is how we live today. As those who suffer from arthritis, perhaps we can appropriate the words of the American freedom song:

**"Deep in my heart, I do believe,
WE SHALL OVERCOME!"**

SOURCES QUOTED

1. Frankl, Viktor E., <u>Man's Search for Meaning</u>, New York: Simon and Schuster, 1959, p. xi.

2. Bonhoeffer, Dietrich<u>, Letters and Papers from Prison</u>. London: SCM Press, 1953, p. 173.

3. Wright, Beatrice A., <u>Physical Disability: A Psychosocial Approach</u>. New York: Harper and Row, 1983, pp. 100-101.

4. Ibid, p. 106.

5. Rosenberg, Alan A., <u>Living With Your Arthritis</u>. New York: Arco Publishing Company, 1979, p. 92.

6. <u>The Holy Bible</u>: Revised Standard Version. New York: Thomas Nelson and Sons, 1952, p. 92.

7. Cousins, Norman, <u>Anatomy of an Illness</u>. New York: Bantam Books, 1981, p. 40.

8. Source unknown.

9. Kubler-Ross, Elisabeth, <u>On Death and Dying</u>. New York: Macmillan Publishing Company, 1969, p. ix.

10. Kushner, Irving, Editor, <u>Understanding Arthritis</u>. New York: Charles Scribner's Sons, 1984, pp. 107—108.

11. Tournier, Paul, <u>Creative Suffering</u>. New York: Harper and Row, 1983, p. 15.

12. Wright, <u>Physical Disability: A Psychosocial Approach</u>. p. 408.

13. Tillich, Paul, <u>Dynamics of Faith</u>. New York: Harper and Row, 1958, p. 111.

14. Pflug, Harold, Editor, <u>Sing To the Lord</u>. Philadelphia: Christian Education Press, 1959, p. 353.

15. Rosenberg, <u>Living With Your Arthritis</u>, p. 132.

16. Wright, <u>Physical Disability: A Psychosocial Approach</u>, pp. 186—187.

SUGGESTED READING

Blau, Sheldon Paul, M.D., <u>Arthritis</u>. Garden City: Doubleday and Company, 1974.

Engleman, Ephraim P., M.D. and Silverman, Milton, Ph.D., <u>The Arthritis Book</u>. Sausalito, California: Painter Hopkins Publishers, 1979.

Fries, James F., M.D., <u>Arthritis</u>. Menlo Park, California: Addison-Wesley Publishing Company, 1979.

Kushner, Irving, Editor, <u>Understanding Arthritis</u>. New York: Charles Scribner's Sons, 1984.

Rosenberg, Alan, M.D., <u>Living With Your Arthritis</u>. New York: Arco Publishing Company, 1979.

MANUALS

Overcoming Rheumatoid Arthritis
Self—Help Manual for Arthritis Patients

PAMPHLETS

Arthritis—The Basic Facts
Aspirin and Related Medications
Gold Treatment
Diet and Nutrition
Inflammation—Unlocking the Mystery
Living and Loving
Practical Information
Quackery and Unproven Remedies
Surgery
Taking Charge: Learning to Live with Arthritis

ARTHRITIS FOUNDATION
1314 Spring Street, N.W.
Atlanta, Georgia 30309

DEAN A. HAUTER, M.D. is a diplomate of the American Board of Family Practice. He is affiliated with the Abraham Lincoln Medical Group in Lincoln, Illinois.

GERSON C. BERNHARD, M.D. is Medical Director of the Midwest Arthritis Treatment Center at Columbia Hospital in Milwaukee and Clinical Professor of Medicine at the Medical College of Wisconsin.

RALPH SEYFERT, who drew the illustrations, was Art Instructor at Homestead High School in Mequon, Wisconsin.

978-0-595-47850-7
0-595-47850-6

www.ingramcontent.com/pod-product-compliance
Lightning Source LLC
Chambersburg PA
CBHW051253050326
40689CB00007B/1175